How To Get GOD'S Attention In Fasting

A Guide To Healthy Fasting

Dr. Vanessa Edwards ND, LAc., MT

How To Get God's Attention In Fasting-A Guide to Healthy Fasting
© 2019 by Dr. Vanessa Edwards.
 All right reserved
Printed in United States of America

Editor: Mrs. Julia Henry
Editor: Elder Johnny Jame

Dr. Vanessa Edwards
Water of Life Naturopathic Healthcare
4421 Salem Ave Dayton OH 45416
www.vedwardsnd.com

Unless otherwise noted, all Scriptures quotations are taken from the King James Version or New American Standard version of the Bible.

ISBN: 13:978-1733561501

The material contained in this book is provided for informational purposes only. It is not intended to diagnose, provide medical advice, or take the place of medical advice and treatment from your physician. Readers are advised to consult with a qualified healthcare professional regarding fasting and/ or treatment of their specific medical problems. The author is not responsible for any possible consequences from any person reading or following the information in this book. If taking prescription medications, consult your physician and do not take yourself off medicines without the proper supervision of a physician.

Dedicated To

My #1 Fan, My Dad
Raymond Edwards

And

My mentor and spiritual mom
Ms. Jannie Wilcoxson
Thank you for teaching me how to study God's word and the importance of fasting. Thank you for leading by example

Hold fast the form of sound words, which thou hast heard of me, in faith and love which is in Christ Jesus   2 Timothy 1:13

CONTENTS

INTRODUCTION

Fasting is a discipline that has been around for centuries. It has been described as one of the most ancient healing traditions in human history. Fasting is practiced by many religions and cultures. Have you ever wondered why this tradition has been around for so long and crossed religious borders?

In the Old Testament of the Bible, the Mosaic Law required fasting only in connection with the observance of the Day of Atonement. Otherwise fasting was voluntary with the exception of fasts proclaimed in times of national emergency.

"This shall be a permanent statute for you: in the seventh month, on the tenth day of the month, you shall humble your souls and not do any work, whether the native, or the alien who sojourns among you; for it is on this day that atonement shall be made for you to cleanse you; you will be clean from all your sins before the LORD. "It is to be a Sabbath of solemn rest for you, that you may humble your souls; it is a permanent statute.

---Leviticus 16:29–31

"On exactly the tenth day of this seventh month is the day of atonement; it shall be a holy convocation for you, and you shall humble your souls and present an offering by fire to the Lord.

---Leviticus 23:27

'Then on the tenth day of this seventh month you shall have a holy convocation, and you shall humble yourselves; you shall not do any work.

---Numbers 29:7

Paul, in the book of Acts, gives us more insight into this Day of Atonement. When he is on a ship headed to Rome, the time of fasting, which refers to the Day of Atonement, was already over.

When considerable time had passed and the

voyage was now dangerous, since even *the fast* was already over, Paul began to admonish them, and said to them, "Men, I perceive that the voyage will certainly be with damage and great loss, not only of the cargo and the ship, but also of our lives.

---Acts 27:9-10

God required Israel to fast once a year on the Day of Atonement, yet we see instances where God was not pleased with their fast. It seems as though the ritual of fasting brought about the idea that if they fasted they would automatically get Gods attention and He would listen to them. For example, in the book of Isaiah, the people inquired of God:

'Why have we fasted and You do not see?

---Isaiah 58:3

Some came to think that fasting would automatically gain God's attention. Against this the prophets declared that without right conduct fasting was in vain.

Fasting has been apart of many different religions and for many different reasons. For instance, the practice of fasting was first very common among the Greeks. The original and most powerful motive for fasting in antiquity was due to fear of demons. It was believed that demons gained power over man through eating. They also believed that fasting was an effective means of preparing for intercourse with deity and for the reception of ecstatic or magical powers. So what makes a believer in the God of the bible and of Jesus Christ, fast different? There seems to be more to getting God's attention while fasting other than just pushing back our forks.

In this study we will take a walk through the scriptures and see how God responded when fasting was initiated. We will look at what actions caused God to react in response to fasting. We will also explore the physical benefits of fasting and how having a lifestyle of fasting may prevent chronic illness.

In Hebrew the word for fasting is *tsoom*, which means to cover the mouth. The Greek word is *nesteuo,* and it means, deliberate and generally prolonged abstention from eating (and sometimes drinking) as a means of humbling oneself before God. There are many documented times of fasting in the Old and New Testament scriptures. We see examples of corporate and individual fasts. In the Christian faith, many times pastors will call for their congregation to participate in corporate fasting. It may be at the beginning of the year, or after a national crisis has occurred. Many times a believer will feel a need to push back their plates when they want to hear God clearly or before they make an important decision. Whatever the reason, when a call to fast is proclaimed it is not just to abstain from food, it is to get God's attention, it is for Him to hear the cry of His people and respond. So how do we get God's attention in fasting?

CHAPTER 1

Does It Matter How Long I Fast?

There are many debates on how long a fast should last. Twenty-one days, or three-week fasts, are very popular, following the example of Daniel, in Daniel 10:2. Also forty day fasts are common, following the example of Jesus in Matthew 4:2. Is it the amount of TIME you spend fasting that gets God's attention? Take a look at the following scriptures and underline the length of time they fasted.

So he *(Moses)* was there with the LORD forty days and forty nights; he did not eat bread or drink water. And he wrote on the tablets the words of the covenant, the Ten Commandments.

----Exodus 34:28

Then David took hold of his clothes and tore them, and *so* also *did* all the men who *were* with him. They mourned and wept and fasted until evening for Saul and his son Jonathan and for the people of the LORD and the house of Israel, because they had fallen by the sword.

----2 Samuel 1:11–12

David therefore inquired of God for the child; and David fasted and went and lay all night on the ground. The elders of his household stood beside him in order to raise him up from the ground, but he was unwilling and would not eat food with them. Then it happened on the seventh day that the child died. So David arose from the ground, washed, anointed *himself,* and changed his clothes; and he came into the house of the LORD and worshiped. Then he came to his own house, and when he requested, they set food before him and he ate.

----2 Samuel 12:16-18, 2

They said to me, "The remnant there in the province who survived the captivity are in great distress and reproach, and the wall of Jerusalem is broken down and its gates are burned with fire." When I heard these words, I sat down and wept and mourned for days; and I was fasting and praying before the God of heaven.

----Nehemiah 1:3–4

And there was a prophetess, Anna the daughter of Phanuel, of the tribe of Asher. She was advanced in years and had lived with *her* husband seven years after her marriage, and then as a widow to the age of eighty-four. She never left the temple, serving night and day with fastings and prayers.

----Luke 2:36

"The Pharisee stood and was praying this to himself: 'God, I thank You that I am not like other people: swindlers, unjust, adulterers, or even like this tax collector. 'I fast twice a week; I pay tithes of all that I get.'

---- Luke 18:11–12

"Whenever you fast, do not put on a gloomy face as the hypocrites *do*, for they neglect their appearance so that they will be noticed by men when they are fasting. Truly I say to you, they have their reward in full.

----Matthew 6:16

Record the lengths of time underlined from the scriptures above:

We see many instances when fasting was instituted and the length of time a person fasted varied. When David mourned the death of Saul and his son, Jonathon, they fasted until evening. When David's son was ill we see him lying on the ground and not eating for seven days, until his son died. Moses was on the mountain with God for forty days with no food or water. The prophetess served in the temple night and day with fasting and prayers. Matthew 6:16 simply states, whenever you fast. There is no set prescription for the length of time a person should fast. And there is no indication that the amount of time you spend fasting will determine whether you will get God's attention or not. So when you sense God calling you to a fast, inquire from Him how long He would like you to abstain.

> So he *(Moses*) was there with the LORD forty days and forty nights; he did not eat bread or drink water. And he wrote on the tablets the words of the covenant, the Ten Commandments.
>
> ----Exodus 34:28

When Moses fasted 40 days and 40 nights, he was in

God's presence. The Lord sustained him. I am not suggesting that you go forty days without food or water, but what I do want you to take from this passage is that Moses spent one on one time with God. It would be of no benefit to your spirit man to set aside time to fast but not set aside time to spend with the Lord. As you are preparing to fast block out specific times to withdraw from your regular routine. Cut off the television, computer, social media, etc. As Pastor Mann says, get off Facebook and put your Face in The Book. Spend time with Jesus. It will be extremely rewarding. This will get God's attention.

CHAPTER 2

When You Fast

In Jesus' Sermon on the Mount, found in the book of Matthew, Jesus is teaching about the basics of righteous living. He sets some parameters for giving, praying and fasting. He warns us not to practice our righteousness before men to be noticed by man. As you read the passage below underline what happens to those who practice righteousness so that others can recognize them. Circle every reference to fasting.

"Beware of practicing your righteousness before

7

men to be noticed by them; otherwise

you have no reward with your Father who is in heaven.

"Whenever you fast, do not put on a gloomy face as the hypocrites do, for they neglect their appearance so that they will be noticed by men when they are fasting. Truly I say to you, they have their reward in full. "But you, when you fast, anoint your head and wash your face so that your fasting will not be noticed by men, but by your Father who is in secret; and your Father who sees what is done in secret will reward you.

---Matthew 6:1, 16–18

When righteousness is practiced to be noticed by man, what is forfeited?

What did you learn from marking the references to

fasting?

How often should we fast?

What should your appearance be like when you fast?

Does it seem like Jesus expects us to fast, according to these scriptures?

Have you ever fasted? If so, describe your experience: length of the fast, what prompted you to fast, what was the outcome?

When You Fast

CHAPTER 3

Jehoshaphat- Do It Afraid

Let's take a look at King Jehoshaphat. He was the son of Asa, king over Judah, during the time Ahab ruled over Israel. He was thirty-five years old when he became king and reigned for twenty-five years in Jerusalem. He had great riches and honor. He followed in his father's footsteps and did right in the sight of the Lord. He removed the high places and the Asherim from Judah. He sent officials and Levites into the cities to teach the law of the Lord to the people. He also made an alliance with the king of Israel, Ahab, by allowing his son to marry Ahab's daughter. This can be found in 1 Kings 22:41-44. During his reign the Moabites and Ammonites, sons of Lot by incestuous union with his daughters, came to make war against him. Draw a circle around every reference to Jehoshaphat.

> Now it came about after this that the sons of Moab and the sons of Ammon, together with some of the Meunites, came to make war against Jehoshaphat. Then some came and reported to Jehoshaphat, saying, "A great multitude is coming against you from beyond the sea, out of Aram and behold, they are in Hazazon-tamar (that is Engedi)." Jehoshaphat was afraid and turned his attention to seek the LORD, and proclaimed a fast throughout all Judah.
>
> ----2 Chronicles 20:1–3

What was Jehoshaphat's reaction to this great multitude that was coming up against him?

How did he respond?

When Jehoshaphat received this news he was afraid of this great multitude coming up against him. While afraid he turned his attention to seek the Lord and proclaimed a fast throughout all Judah. Many will say that fear and faith cannot occur at the same time. They will say, if you have fear, you have no faith. In many instances this may be true but we see something totally different in this passage. The indicator of faith is not whether or not you have fear. Fear is a natural and physical response to danger. God created us that way. When our brain detects danger, it immediately responds by producing epinephrine and norepinephrine. These neurotransmitters are known as the "fight or flight neurotransmitters", they help us realize that danger is near and gives us the ability to either stay and fight our way out of a negative situation or flight...get the heck out of dodge. So if being afraid is not the indicator of whether or not you have faith in a situation, then what is the indicator? The answer is found in verse three. When Jehoshaphat was afraid, he turned his attention to seek the Lord, and proclaimed a fast. It was his response; he is looking to the Lord and expecting an answer. If we let fear paralyze us and don't turn to God, that would be a lack of faith, but if we seek Him in the midst of our fear as Jehoshaphat did, we posses faith and we are doing it afraid. Another example of doing it afraid in the scriptures is when the Philistines capture David in Gath. Read his response:

> Be gracious to me, O God, for man has trampled upon me; fighting all day long he oppresses me. My foes have trampled upon me all day long, for they are many who fight proudly against me. When I am afraid, I will put my trust in You. In God, whose word I praise, In God I have put my trust; I shall not be afraid. What can mere man do to me?

> ----Psalm 56:1–4

What does David do when he is afraid?

How do you respond when you are afraid?

Back to Jehoshaphat:

The king proclaimed a corporate fast. All the inhabitants of Judah, including infants, wives, and children, began to gather from all the cities and began to seek help from the Lord. Jehoshaphat went to the house of the Lord, where they were assembled and began to pray. Let's take a look at his prayer. Underline all references to God, including you and your.

And he said, "O LORD, the God of our fathers, are You not God in the heavens? And are You not ruler over all the kingdoms of the nations? Power and might are in Your hand so that no one can stand against You. "Did You not, O our God, drive out the inhabitants of this land before Your people Israel and give it to the descendants of Abraham Your friend forever? "They have lived in it, and have built You a sanctuary there for Your name, saying, 'Should evil come upon us, the sword, or judgment, or pestilence, or famine, we will stand before this house and before You (for Your name is in this house) and cry to You in our distress, and You will hear and deliver us.' "Now behold, the sons of Ammon and Moab and Mount Seir, whom You did not let Israel invade when they came out of the land of Egypt (they turned aside from them and did not destroy them), see how they are rewarding us by coming to drive us out from Your possession which You have given us as an inheritance. "O our God, will You not judge them? For we are powerless before this great multitude who are coming against us; nor do we know what to do, but our eyes are on You."

----2 Chronicles 20:6–12

How did Jehoshaphat describe God?

What did the forefather's say they would do if evil came upon them?

How did they believe God would respond?

Who gave them possession of the land?

How does Jehoshaphat describe their position?

Jehoshaphat is exalting God for who He is...God of our fathers, the creator of the heavens, and ruler of all kingdoms. So powerful that power and might are in His hand and no one has the ability to stand against Him. Then he begins to remind God of what He did and what He said....You drove out the inhabitants of this land, you said this land was to be given to Abraham and his descendants forever. Therefore, they came and settled in the land that you gave them. They built homes, and communities; they even built a sanctuary for you. You said that this land is our inheritance, now the enemy is trying to take possession of what you said belongs to us. Jehoshaphat **is praying back to God what He said.** Lord, you said... We should take some notes, and pray scripture back to God when we find ourselves in an impossible situation. For example, in times of need...Lord you said you would supply all my needs according to your riches in glory. Times when you feel anxious...Lord you said that I should be anxious for nothing but by prayer and supplication let my request be made known unto you; therefore I am choosing to trust you with this situation. When you feel alone...Lord your word says, You will never leave me nor forsaken me, therefore; I choose not to be swayed by my emotions but to believe your word.

Jehoshaphat recognized God's power and authority. He also recognized their lack of power without God. He proceeds to tell God, in his prayer, we don't know what to do, but our eyes are on You. Remember, this is the king, praying in front of all of Judah admitting that he is helpless, admitting that he does not know what to do to protect the people from this very present danger. This takes humility. What a great position to be in, total dependence on God. Have you ever been here? There is nothing more you can do, say, no one to call to fix the problem. If it is going to be fixed, God has to do it. My mentor, Jannie Wilcoxson, called this, miracle territory.

This is where God wants us, our eyes on Him. When I travel to other countries doing missions, often times we see miracles occur right before our very eyes. The question is often asked, why don't we see more miracles in America? The answer maybe, we have too many options, and most of the time God is not our first choice.

Let's look at the passage and see how God responds. The people are fasting, they have gathered at the house of God, they have prayed God's word back to Him, they have reminded Him of His promises and they are totally dependent upon God. Read the passage below, underline all references to Lord/God and record how God responds.

All Judah was standing before the LORD, with their infants, their wives and their children.

Then in the midst of the assembly the Spirit of the LORD came upon Jahaziel the son of Zechariah, the son of Benaiah, the son of Jeiel, the son of Mattaniah, the Levite of the sons of Asaph; and he said, "Listen, all Judah and the inhabitants of Jerusalem and King Jehoshaphat: thus says the LORD to you, 'Do not fear or be dismayed because of this great multitude, for the battle is not yours but God's. 'Tomorrow go down against them. Behold, they will come up by the ascent of Ziz, and you will find them at the end of the valley in front of the wilderness of Jeruel. 'You need not fight in this battle; station yourselves, stand and see the salvation of the LORD on your behalf, O Judah and Jerusalem.' Do not fear or be dismayed; tomorrow go out to face them, for the LORD is with you." Jehoshaphat bowed his head with his face to the ground, and all Judah and the inhabitants of Jerusalem fell down before the LORD, worshiping the LORD. The Levites, from the sons of the Kohathites and of the sons of the Korahites, stood up to praise the LORD God of Israel, with a very loud voice.

----2 Chronicles 20:13–19

Who did the Lord speak through?

What was God's message?

What were God's instructions?

Did fasting, praying, humbling oneself, and seeking God for direction, get God's attention?

They listened to God, rose early the next morning and went to the wilderness of Tekoa. Jehoshaphat encouraged them to put their trust in God and God would establish them. He also encouraged them to put their trust in God's prophets and they would succeed. He then had the singers to begin singing praises unto the

Lord and as they sang, the Lord set an ambush against the Ammonites, Moabites, and the inhabitants of Mount Seir. They then turned on one another and they were all destroyed. When Judah arrived there was nothing left but dead bodies, no one escaped.

Benefits/ Blessings of participating in corporate fasting

Continuing with the passage in 2 Chronicles 20

> When Jehoshaphat and his people came to take their spoil, they found much among them, including goods, garments and valuable things which they took for themselves, more than they could carry. And they were three days taking the spoil because there was so much. Then on the fourth day they assembled in the valley of Beracah, for there they blessed the LORD. Therefore they have named that place "The Valley of Beracah" until today. Every man of Judah and Jerusalem returned with Jehoshaphat at their head, returning to Jerusalem with joy, for the

LORD had made them to rejoice over their enemies. They came to Jerusalem with harps, lyres and trumpets to the house of the LORD. And the dread of God was on all the kingdoms of the lands when they heard that the LORD had fought against the enemies of Israel. So the kingdom of Jehoshaphat was at peace, for his God gave him rest on all sides.

----2 Chronicles 20:25–30

What did the people find?

How much did they find?

How many days did it take for them to collect the spoil?

What did the other kingdoms hear?

What did the other kingdoms experience?

What did Jehoshaphat and Judah experience?

When Judah united by fasting, praying, humbling themselves and seeking God, they got God's attention.

Not only did God fight for them, and the enemy was annihilated without them having to fight, he also blessed them. There were so many valuable things that they acquired from the enemy, that it took three days to collect it all. There was an overflow of blessings. The word also spread to all the other kingdoms and they were put on notice, don't mess with God's people. They no longer had to worry about the enemy coming up against them, God gave them peace and rest on all sides.

Just as God had a purpose and plan for Jehosophat, the king of Judah's, life. God also has a plan and purpose for your life. When you are faced with an impossible situation do you fast, humble yourself, seek God and pray? God will hear you and answer you. He will not allow the enemy to overtake you. He will fight your battles for you and you will find an overflow of blessings, peace and rest, in Him. Remember you are His child. Jeremiah 29:11 says, for I know the plans that I have for you,' declares the LORD, 'plans for welfare and not for calamity to give you a future and a hope.

CHAPTER 4

Joel-Your Whole Heart

Let's take a look at the writings of Joel. We don't know much about this writer. Let's look at what we do know. Joel's name means "Jehovah is God". He was a prophet, he prophesied during the rule of Joash, king of the southern kingdom. 2 Kings 11 and 12 gives us some insight on what the climate was like during Joel's time.

Joash became king at the age of 7 years old. He was appointed king after his grandmother stole the throne by killing all the royal offspring after the death of her son, so she could become queen. Wow! How could a grandma kill her own grandkids? Joash was hidden and raised in the same house as Queen Athaliah for six years. In the 7th year the priest, Jehoiada revealed Joash to the people and he was crowned king. Grandma, Queen Athaliah was put to death. Even in this chaos, God had a plan.

King Joash reigned 40 years in Jerusalem and did right in the sight of the Lord as long as Jehoiada, the priest, was alive, yet the people still sacrificed and burned incense on the high places. A little history. In Numbers 34:52, God gave specific instructions to Israel, through Moses, to destroy all the molten images and to demolish all their high places, when they came into Canaan.

During King Joash's reign the house of the Lord was repaired. Priest Jehoiada died at a ripe old age of 130. After his death king Joash began to listen to the officials of Judah. Read the passage below, 2 Chronicles 24:17-19, twice. Underline what the king and the people did, reread and then circle God's response.

> But after the death of Jehoiada the officials of
> Judah came and bowed down to the king, and the

king listened to them. They (Judah) abandoned the house of the LORD, the God of their fathers, and served the Asherim and the idols; so wrath came upon Judah and Jerusalem for this their guilt. Yet He (God) sent prophets to them (Judah) to bring them back to the LORD; though they (the prophets) testified against them, they (Judah) would not listen.

----2Chronicals 24:17-19

Did the king receive wise counsel from the officials?

What did the people do?

What was God's response?

Who did God send to bring them back to Himself?

Joel was among these prophets. A plague had come to Judah. Read the passage in Joel 1 to get insight on what was occurring during this time. Underline all references to elders and inhabitants of the land.

> The word of the LORD that came to Joel, the son of Pethuel: Hear this, O elders, and listen, all inhabitants of the land. Has anything like this happened in your days or in your fathers' days? Tell your sons about it, and let your sons tell their sons, and their sons the next generation. What the gnawing locust has left, the swarming locust has eaten; and what the swarming locust has left, the creeping locust

has eaten; And what the creeping locust has left, the stripping locust has eaten. Awake, drunkards, and weep; And wail, all you wine drinkers, On account of the sweet wine that is cut off from your mouth. For a nation has invaded my land, mighty and without number; its teeth are the teeth of a lion, and it has the fangs of a lioness. It has made my vine a waste and my fig tree splinters. It has stripped them bare and cast them away; their branches have become white.

---- Joel 1:1–7

What was happening in Judah?

What is Joel suggesting they do?

Who or what is causing turmoil?

Judah was experiencing a great famine. A great nation had come up against them and invaded the land. Joel is encouraging them to pass this information on for generations to come. He is encouraging them to wake up! In the next passage, underline who/ what is affected by this famine.

Wail like a virgin girded with sackcloth, for the bridegroom of her youth. The grain offering and the drink offering are cut off from the house of the LORD. The priests mourn, the ministers of the LORD. The field is ruined, the land mourns; for the grain is ruined, the new wine dries up, fresh oil fails. Be ashamed, O farmers, Wail, O vinedressers, for the wheat and the barley; because the harvest of the field is destroyed. The vine dries up and the fig tree fails; the pomegranate, the palm also, and the apple tree, all the trees of the field dry up. Indeed, rejoicing dries up from the sons of men.

---- Joel 1:8–12

Record who/what is affected by this famine

The famine affected all, nothing and no one was exempt. From the leaders, to the land, to the people, there was no rejoicing in the land. In the following passage, underline each reference to priests and ministers.

Gird yourselves with sackcloth and lament, O priests; Wail, O ministers of the altar! Come; spend the night in sackcloth O ministers of my God, for the grain offering and the drink offering are withheld from the house of your God. Consecrate a fast, proclaim a solemn assembly; gather the elders and all the inhabitants of the land to the house of the LORD your God, and cry out to the LORD. Alas for the day! For the day of the LORD is near, and it will come as destruction from the Almighty. Has not food been cut off before our eyes, Gladness and joy from the house of our God? The seeds shrivel under their clods; the storehouses are desolate, the barns are torn down, for the grain is dried up.

----Joel 1:13–17

Who is he talking to?

What does Joel suggest they do?

Joel urges the leaders, the priest and ministers, to put on sackcloth, to lament and wail. Putting on sackcloth is a

sign of humbling oneself. The famine is so bad they
aren't even able to make a drink or grain sacrifice to God.
He encourages them to gather everyone, to the house of
the Lord, fast corporately and cry out to God.
Devastation is upon them. God is the only one that can
deliver them. Joel is encouraging them to return to God.
Underline every reference to God/Lord.

"Yet even now," declares the LORD, "Return to Me with all your heart, And with fasting, weeping and mourning; and rend your heart and not your garments." Now return to the LORD your God, for He is gracious and compassionate, slow to anger, abounding in lovingkindness and relenting of evil. Who knows whether He will *not* turn and relent and leave a blessing behind Him, *even* a grain offering and a drink offering for the LORD your God? Blow a trumpet in Zion, Consecrate a fast, proclaim a solemn assembly, gather the people, sanctify the congregation, assemble the elders, gather the children and the nursing infants. Let the bridegroom come out of his room and the bride out of her *bridal* chamber. Let the priests, the LORD's ministers, weep between the porch and the altar, and let them say, "Spare Your people, O LORD, and do not make Your inheritance a reproach, A byword among the nations. Why should they among the peoples say, 'Where is their God?' "

---- Joel 2:12 -17

How does the Lord want them to return to Him?

They were tearing their cloths and putting on sackcloth, what does the Lord want them to rend?

What attributes of God are discussed in this passage?

Who does he want to participate?

The Lord wants their heart, their whole heart. Everyone is called to participate in giving his or her hearts back to the Lord. Everyone is called to fast, and return to the Lord, from the priests, ministers, elders, to the children, nursing infants, and even newlyweds. Joel says, He may relent and leave a blessing behind Him. This may get God's attention. We see a similar situation in the book of Revelation; the church of Ephesus had left their first love, God. They were encouraged to repent and return to Him.

In these passages, Joel isn't speaking to the world, those without God. He is speaking to God's chosen people. He is encouraging them to repent from their wicked ways and follow Him. Are we, the church, the ecclesia of God, the called out ones in need of repentance? Do we need to rend our hearts and not just our clothes? Have we left our first love? Are we letting things of the world take precedent over our God?   Can we truly say God is pleased with the body of Christ? Do we need to return with **fasting**, weeping, and mourning? Is God using tragedy and devastating events to get our attention? Are we paying attention?

God's response to their praying, fasting, and repentant heart:

Underline all references to Lord in the passage.

> Then the LORD will be zealous for His land and will have pity on His people.
>
> The LORD will answer and say to His people, "Behold, I am going to send you   grain, new wine and oil, and you will be satisfied in full with them; And I will never again make you a reproach among the nations. "Then I will make up to you for the years that the swarming locust has eaten, the creeping locust, the stripping locust and the gnawing locust, my great army which I sent among you. "You will have plenty to eat and be satisfied and praise the name of the LORD your God, Who has dealt wondrously with you; Then My

people will never be put to shame. "Thus you will know that I am in the midst of Israel, and that I am the LORD your God, and there is no other; and My people will never be put to shame.

----Joel 2:18–19, 25-27

What did you learn from marking the word Lord?

Will His people have to go through some tough times?

Will the Lord deliver them?

Who will make up for the years devastated by locust?

God responded to their prayers, their fasting, their repentant heart. This got God's attention.

CHAPTER 5

Ezra-Protection

In the book of Ezra, the children of Israel had been in exile in Babylon for 70 years. The Medes and Persian empire grew strong and they defeated Babylon. Under the rule of Cyrus, the king of Persia, any Jewish person willing to go back and rebuild the temple was allowed to return to Jerusalem.

Now in the first year of Cyrus king of Persia, in order to fulfill the word of the LORD by the mouth of Jeremiah, the LORD stirred up the spirit of Cyrus king of Persia, so that he sent a proclamation throughout all his kingdom, and also put it in writing, saying: "Thus says Cyrus king of Persia, 'The LORD, the God of heaven, has given me all the kingdoms of the earth and He has appointed me to build Him a house in Jerusalem, which is in Judah. 'Whoever there is among you of all His people, may his God be with him! Let him go up to Jerusalem which is in Judah and rebuild the house of the LORD, the God of Israel; He is the God who is in Jerusalem.

----Ezra 1:1–3

Who did God use to prophesy about the return of Israel to Jerusalem?

Why did King Cyrus issue a proclamation to allow the Jews to return to Jerusalem?

Who did King Cyrus give credit to for giving him all the kingdoms of the earth?

What was Cyrus appointed to do?

What were the people to do once they returned?

Let's take a look at Jeremiah's prophecy.   Underline each reference to Lord in the passage.

> "For thus says the LORD, 'When seventy years have been completed for Babylon, I will visit you and fulfill My good word to you, to bring you back to this place.

> --
>
> --Jeremiah 29:10

What time period had to be completed in Babylon?

What was Jeremiah's prophecy?

Judah had been in captivity , to Babylon, for seventy years because of their disobedience. One of the statutes they broke was not allowing the land to have a Sabbath rest. They were suppose to allow the land to rest, grow no food, every seventh year. They ignored this ordinance for 70 years. The repercussions for not obeying God was that they would spend 70 years, 1 year for every Sabbath missed, in captivity.

The following passage will give you insight on what they were doing when they returned to Israel.

> Now in the second year of their coming to the house of God at Jerusalem in the second month, Zerubbabel the son of Shealtiel and Jeshua the son of Jozadak and the rest of their brothers the priests and the Levites, and all who came from the captivity to Jerusalem, began *the work and* appointed the Levites from twenty years and older to oversee the work of the house of the LORD.
>
> Then Jeshua with his sons and brothers stood united with Kadmiel and his sons, the sons of Judah and the sons of Henadad with their sons and brothers the Levites, to oversee the

workmen in the temple of God. Now when the builders had laid the foundation of the temple of the LORD, the priests stood in their apparel with trumpets, and the Levites, the sons of Asaph, with cymbals, to praise the LORD according to the directions of King David of Israel. They sang, praising and giving thanks to the LORD, saying, "For He is good, for His lovingkindness is upon Israel forever." And all the people shouted with a great shout when they praised the LORD because the foundation of the house of the LORD was laid. Yet many of the priests and Levites and heads of fathers' households, the old men who had seen the first temple, wept with a loud voice when the foundation of this house was laid before their eyes, while many shouted aloud for joy, so that the people could not distinguish the sound of the shout of joy from the sound of the weeping of the people, for the people shouted with a loud shout, and the sound was heard far away.

----Ezra 3:8–13

When did they begin to work on the house of the Lord?

What was their reaction once the foundation was laid?

What was the reaction of those who had seen the first temple?

Underline all references to the enemies of Judah and Benjamin.

> Now when the enemies of Judah and Benjamin heard that the people of the exile were building a temple to the LORD God of Israel, they approached Zerubbabel and the heads of fathers' households, and said to them, "Let us

build with you, for we, like you, seek your God; and we have been sacrificing to Him since the days of Esarhaddon king of Assyria, who brought us up here." But Zerubbabel and Jeshua and the rest of the heads of fathers' households of Israel said to them, "You have nothing in common with us in building a house to our God; but we ourselves will together build to the LORD God of Israel, as King Cyrus, the king of Persia has commanded us." Then the people of the land discouraged the people of Judah, and frightened them from building, and hired counselors against them to frustrate their counsel all the days of Cyrus king of Persia, even until the reign of Darius king of Persia.

----Ezra 4:1–5

What was the enemy's first approach?

Since "being friendly" didn't work, what did they try next?

Be careful whom you allow to join in on the vision that God has given you. They were not swayed by the sweet talk of the enemy; they did not allow them to participate in the building of the temple. Since that didn't work, the enemy had another strategy, discouragement and fear. They spent large sums of money to hire counselors to frustrate their plans. The counselors were put on staff during the reign of Cyrus to the reign of Darius. Cyrus reigned from 539BC to 530BC. Darius began his reign in 521BC. The enemy is always on his job, he doesn't take a break. The building of the temple was delayed for 14 years because the enemy instilled fear and discouragement into the people of Judah. It is critical that you know your assignment. When you are sure of your assignment, this will help you stand in the midst of adversity. Opposition doesn't mean God isn't in it.

In Ezra chapter 5, the prophets Haggai and Zechariah began to prophesy to the people. They had to recast the vision, get them back on track, so that they would resume the building of the temple, despite the opposition.

When the prophets, Haggai the prophet and Zechariah the son of Iddo, prophesied to the Jews who were in Judah and Jerusalem in the name of the God of Israel, who was over them, then Zerubbabel the son of Shealtiel and Jeshua the son of Jozadak arose and began to rebuild the house of God which is in Jerusalem; and the prophets of God were with them supporting them.

----Ezra 5:1–2

Once they got back on track, and began to rebuild the temple, the enemy appeared again. Underline God's response.

> At that time Tattenai, the governor of the province beyond the River, and Shethar-bozenai

and their colleagues came to them and spoke to them thus, "Who issued you a decree to rebuild this temple and to finish this structure?" Then we told them accordingly what the names of the men were who were reconstructing this building. But the eye of their God was on the elders of the Jews, and they did not stop them until a report could come to Darius, and then a written reply be returned concerning it.

----Ezra 5:3-5

What did the governor and his colleagues ask them?

What was the people's response?

What was God's position?

The construction of the temple continued. A letter was sent by the governor of the province to King Darius, who reigned with and after Cyrus King of Persia, to stop the rebuilding of the temple. Read the contents of the letter below, underline their request.

> This is the copy of the letter which Tattenai, the governor of the province beyond the River, and Shethar-bozenai and his colleagues the officials, who were beyond the River, sent to Darius the king.
> They sent a report to him in which it was written thus: "To Darius the king, all peace.
> "Let it be known to the king that we have gone to the province of Judah, to the house of the great God, which is being built with huge stones, and beams are being laid in the walls; and this work is going on with great care and is succeeding in their hands.
>
> "Then we asked those elders and said to them thus, 'Who issued you a decree to rebuild this temple and to finish this structure?'
> "We also asked them their names so as to inform you, and that we might write down the

names of the men who were at their head.

"Thus they answered us, saying, 'We are the servants of the God of heaven and earth and are rebuilding the temple that was built many years ago, which a great king of Israel built and finished.

'But because our fathers had provoked the God of heaven to wrath, He gave them into the hand of Nebuchadnezzar king of Babylon, the Chaldean, who destroyed this temple and deported the people to Babylon.

'However, in the first year of Cyrus king of Babylon, King Cyrus issued a decree to rebuild this house of God.

'Also the gold and silver utensils of the house of God which Nebuchadnezzar had taken from the temple in Jerusalem, and brought them to the temple of Babylon, these King Cyrus took from the temple of Babylon and they were given to one whose name was Sheshbazzar, whom he had appointed governor. 'He said to him, "Take these utensils, go and deposit them in the temple in Jerusalem and let the house of God be rebuilt in its place. 'Then that Sheshbazzar came and laid the foundations of the house of God in Jerusalem; and from then until now it has been under construction and it is not yet completed.' "Now if it pleases the king, let a search be conducted in the king's treasure house, which is there in Babylon, if it be that a decree was issued by King Cyrus to rebuild this house of God at Jerusalem; and let the king send to us his decision concerning this matter."

----Ezra 5: 6-17

Below is the response of King Darius:

Then King Darius issued a decree, and search was made in the archives, where the treasures were stored in Babylon. In Ecbatana in the fortress, which is in the province of Media, a scroll was found and there was written in it as follows:

"Memorandum— "In the first year of King Cyrus, Cyrus the king issued a decree: 'Concerning the house of God at Jerusalem, let the temple, the place where sacrifices are offered, be rebuilt and let its foundations be retained, its height being 60 cubits and its width 60 cubits; with three layers of huge stones and one layer of timbers. And let the cost be paid from the royal treasury. 'Also let the gold and silver utensils of the house of God, which Nebuchadnezzar took from the temple in Jerusalem and brought to Babylon, be returned and brought to their places in the temple in Jerusalem; and you shall put them in the house of God.' "Now therefore, Tattenai, governor of the province beyond the River, Shethar-bozenai and your colleagues, the officials of the provinces beyond the River, keep away from there. "Leave this work on the house of God alone; let the governor of the Jews and the elders of the Jews rebuild this house of God on its site. "Moreover, I issue a decree concerning what you are to do for these elders of Judah in the rebuilding of this house of God: the full cost is to be paid to these people from the royal treasury out of the taxes of the provinces beyond the River, and that without delay. "Whatever is needed, both young bulls, rams, and lambs for a burnt offering to the God of heaven, and wheat, salt, wine and anointing oil, as the priests in Jerusalem request, it is to be given to them daily without fail, that they may offer acceptable sacrifices to the God of heaven and pray for the life of the king and his sons. "And I issued a decree that any man who violates this edict, a timber shall be drawn from his house and he shall be impaled on it and his house shall be made a refuse heap on account of this.

"May the God who has caused His name to dwell there overthrow any king or people who attempts to change it, so as to destroy this house of God in Jerusalem. I, Darius, have issued this decree, let it be carried out with all diligence!" Then Tattenai, the governor of the province beyond the River, Shethar-bozenai and their colleagues carried out the decree with all diligence, just as King Darius had sent.

----Ezra 6:1–13

What were the orders given by King Darius to the governor of the province, Tattnenai?

What did King Darius command the enemy to do for

the elders of Judah in the rebuilding of God's house?

What would happen to anyone who violated this edict?

What the enemy meant for evil, God worked it out for their good. When opposition arises, continue to stand in spite of it. Continue to press toward the mark of the high calling in Christ Jesus our Lord. God has given you an assignment and He has given you the ability and resources to complete the assignment in the midst of opposition.

We finally get to Ezra in chapter 7

> Now after these things, in the reign of Artaxerxes king of Persia, there went up Ezra son of Seraiah, son of Azariah, son of Hilkiah, son of Shallum, son of Zadok, son of Ahitub, son of Amariah, son of Azariah, son of Meraioth, son of Zerahiah, son of Uzzi, son of Bukki, son of Abishua, son of Phinehas, son of Eleazar, son of Aaron the chief priest. This Ezra went up from Babylon, and he was a scribe skilled in the law of Moses, which the LORD God of Israel had given; and the king granted him all he requested because the hand of the LORD his God was upon him. Some of the sons of Israel and some of the priests, the Levites, the singers, the gatekeepers and the temple servants went up to Jerusalem in the seventh year of King Artaxerxes. He came to Jerusalem in the fifth month, which was in the seventh year of the king. For on the first of the first month he began to go up from Babylon; and on the first of the fifth month he came to Jerusalem, because the good hand of his God was upon him. For Ezra had set his heart to study the law of the LORD and to practice it, and to teach His statutes and ordinances in Israel.

----Ezra 7:1–10

What is the time period?

Where was Ezra?

What was his occupation?

Why did the king grant him favor?

When did Ezra go to Jerusalem?

Ezra didn't return to Jerusalem with the first set of Israelites, during Cyrus's reign. Yet when he did return, he returned with a purpose. What had he set his heart to do in verse 10?

Underline the ordinances found in the decree:

Now this is the copy of the decree which King Artaxerxes gave to Ezra the priest, the scribe, learned in the words of the commandments of the LORD and His statutes to Israel:

"Artaxerxes, king of kings, to Ezra the priest, the scribe of the law of the God of heaven, perfect peace. And now I have issued a decree that any of the people of Israel and their priests and the Levites in my kingdom who are willing to go to Jerusalem, may go with you. "Forasmuch as you are sent by the king and his seven counselors to inquire concerning Judah and Jerusalem according to the law of your God which is in your hand, and to bring the silver and gold, which the king and his counselors have freely offered to the God of Israel, whose dwelling is in Jerusalem, with all the silver and gold which you find in the whole province of Babylon, along with the freewill offering of the people and of the priests, who offered willingly for the house of their God which is in Jerusalem; with this money, therefore, you shall diligently buy bulls, rams and lambs, with their grain offerings and their drink offerings and offer them on the altar of the house of your God which is in Jerusalem. "Whatever seems good to you and to your brothers to do with the rest of the silver and gold, you may do according to the will of your God. "Also the utensils which are given to you for the service of the house of your God, deliver in full before the God of Jerusalem.

"The rest of the needs for the house of your God, for which you may have occasion to "I, even I, King Artaxerxes, issue a decree to all the treasurers who are in the provinces beyond the River, that whatever Ezra the priest, the scribe of the law of the God of heaven, may require of you, it shall be done diligently, even up to 100 talents of silver, 100 kors of wheat, 100 baths of wine, 100 baths of oil, and salt as needed.

"Whatever is commanded by the God of heaven, let it be done with zeal for the house of the God of heaven, so that there will not be wrath against the kingdom of the king and his sons.

"We also inform you that it is not allowed to impose tax, tribute or toll on any of the priests, Levites, singers, doorkeepers, Nethinim or servants of this house of God. "You, Ezra, according to the wisdom of your God which is in your hand, appoint magistrates and judges that they may judge all the people who are in the province beyond the River, even all those who know the laws of your God; and you may teach anyone who is ignorant of them. "Whoever will not observe the law of your God and the law of the king, let judgment be executed upon him strictly, whether for death or for banishment or for confiscation of goods or for imprisonment."

----Ezra 7:11–26

Who could return to Israel in the decree issued by King Artaxerxes?

What was Ezra to take with him?

What were they to do with the money?

What would happen to those who didn't observe the law?

Put a circle around the word Ezra, below, and any references to him:

> Blessed be the LORD, the God of our fathers, who
> has put such a thing as this in the king's heart,
> to adorn the house of the LORD which is in
> Jerusalem, and has extended lovingkindness to

me before the king and his counselors and before all the king's mighty princes. Thus I was strengthened according to the hand of the LORD my God upon me, and I gathered leading men from Israel to go up with me.

---Ezra 7:27–28

What was Ezra's response?

Who put this idea in the king's heart?

Where did Ezra get the strength to carry out the task?

Once again circle the word Ezra and any references to him:

> Then I proclaimed a fast there at the river of Ahava, that we might humble ourselves before our God to seek from Him a safe journey for us, our little ones, and all our possessions. For I was ashamed to request from the king troops and horsemen to protect us from the enemy on the way, because we had said to the king, "The hand of our God is favorably disposed to all those who seek Him, but His power and His anger are against all those who forsake Him." So we fasted and sought our God concerning this matter, and He listened to our entreaty.

> ----Ezra 8:21–23

What did Ezra do?

Why did he proclaim a fast?

What was God's response?

 Ezra was strengthened, by the hand of the Lord, to carry out a task that could have cost him his life. He and many others, including women and children would be traveling from Babylon to Jerusalem with great possessions, silver, gold, and money.   This was a very dangerous assignment. He was ashamed to ask the king for protection because he had bragged about how God would protect them, so he proclaimed a **fast** at the river Ahava. They humbled themselves and asked God for a safe journey for themselves and the little ones and their possessions. And God heard and answered their prayers.

Have you ever been given an assignment by God and you thought, I can't do this, do you really want me to do this God, Lord are you sure you have the right person?   Your assignment may not cost you your physical life, but will take much dying to self. When we are faced with these situations it would be good to take a lesson from Ezra and push back our plates, seek God, humble ourselves and ask Him for protection and direction. He will hear and answer.

CHAPTER 6

Ahab and Jezebel- False Fast

The next person we are going to study is Ahab. First we will get some background on Ahab and then see what we can learn from him.   Underline all references to Ahab.

Now Ahab the son of Omri became king over Israel in the thirty-eighth year of Asa king of

Judah, and Ahab the son of Omri reigned over Israel in Samaria twenty-two years. Ahab the son of Omri did evil in the sight of the LORD more than all who were before him. It came about, as though it had been a trivial thing for him to walk in the sins of Jeroboam the son of Nebat, that he married Jezebel the daughter of Ethbaal king of the Sidonians, and went to serve Baal and worshiped him. So he erected an altar for Baal in the house of Baal which he built in Samaria. Ahab also made the Asherah. Thus Ahab did more to provoke the LORD God of Israel than all the kings of Israel who were before him.

---1 Kings 16:29–33

Surely there was no one like Ahab who sold himself to do evil in the sight of the LORD, because Jezebel his wife incited him.

---1 Kings 21:25

What was Ahab's position?

How long did he reign?

What did Ahab do to provoke the Lord?

Who did he marry?

How does the writer describe Ahab?

What gods did he serve and worship?

Ahab's decision to worship Baal influenced the people of Israel. God was not pleased with this. God used Elijah to challenge the people to choose between God and Baal, on Mt. Carmel. "How long will you hesitate between two opinions? If the Lord is God, follow him, but if Baal, follow him, 1 Kings 18:21." Elijah had the prophets of Baal choose an oxen and lay it on the alter for a sacrifice to Baal. If Baal were a true god he would provide fire to burn the sacrifice. The prophets of Baal, called on Baal from morning until evening, and there was no answer. While they called on Baal, Elijah mocked them, saying things like, "call him a little louder, maybe he can't hear you, maybe he went on a journey or is asleep". They called louder, and even cut themselves, but there was no answer. It was now Elijah's turn. Read the passage and underline God's response.

> Then Elijah said to all the people, "Come near to me." So all the people came near to him. And he repaired the altar of the LORD which had been torn down. Elijah took twelve stones

according to the number of the tribes of the sons of Jacob, to whom the word of the LORD had come, saying, "Israel shall be your name." So with the stones he built an altar in the name of the LORD, and he made a trench around the altar, large enough to hold two measures of seed. Then he arranged the wood and cut the ox in pieces and laid *it* on the wood. And he said, "Fill four pitchers with water and pour *it* on the burnt offering and on the wood." And he said, "Do it a second time," and they did it a second time. And he said, "Do it a third time," and they did it a third time. The water flowed around the altar and he also filled the trench with water. At the time of the offering of the evening sacrifice, Elijah the prophet came near and said, "O LORD, the God of Abraham, Isaac and Israel, today let it be known that You are God in Israel and that I am Your servant and I have done all these things at Your word. "Answer me, O LORD, answer me, that this people may know that You, O LORD, are God, and that You have turned their heart back again." Then the fire of the LORD fell and consumed the burnt offering and the wood and the stones and the dust, and licked up the water that was in the trench. When all the people saw it, they fell on their faces; and they said, "The LORD, He is God; the LORD, He is God."

---1 Kings 18:30–39

There is no mention of fasting in this passage but Elijah definitely got God's attention.

What did Elijah add to the altar that the prophets of Baal didn't have?

How did God respond?

How did the people respond?

Ok, now back to Ahab. Ahab goes to speak to his neighbor Naboth about purchasing his vineyard. He wanted to buy it so that he could plant a vegetable garden, close to his house. Read the passage below to see how Naboth responds and how Ahab responds.

> But Naboth said to Ahab, "The LORD forbid me
> that I should give you the inheritance of my
> fathers." So Ahab came into his house sullen and
> vexed because of the word which Naboth the
> Jezreelite had spoken to him; for he said, "I will
> not give you the inheritance of my fathers." And
> he lay down on his bed and turned away his face
> and ate no food.

---1 Kings 21:3–4

Word Study

Sullen-definition: stubborn, resentful, implacable

Vexed- definition: raging, great displeasure

What was Naboth's response?

What was Ahab's response?

Naboth was in a tough position. The king of Israel came to him personally and asked to purchase his land. He may have been tempted to sale, after all, it was the king and I'm sure the king offered to compensate him well. Naboth had to choose between pleasing the King of Israel and the King of Kings. His reason for not selling the land was because the Lord would not allow him to sale it. In Numbers 36:7, it states that "Thus no inheritance of the sons of Israel shall be transferred from tribe to tribe, for the sons of Israel shall each hold to the inheritance of the tribe of his fathers. Naboth chose to follow God. This decision did not sit well with the king. He was so upset that he went to bed and wouldn't eat anything. Now, this is not an example of a fast that would get God's attention. He is all in his feelings. He is so depressed because he couldn't get what he wanted, because someone said no to him that he won't even eat.

Have you ever been so down and depressed over a situation that you just couldn't do anything. You don't pray, seek God, or godly counsel and the thought of food just makes things worse. Well, this type of fast probably won't get God to move on your behalf.

In 1 Kings 21: 8-13, Ahab was so upset that when his wife, Jezebel, saw him she asked him why he was so down in his spirit and not eating. He then shared the conversation that he had with Naboth, with her. She responds to him by basically saying, "aren't you the king", don't worry honey; I will take care of it. Get up out of this bed, let your heart be joyful and eat! The passage below tells how she handles it. Underline the information contained in the letter written by Jezebel:

So she wrote letters in Ahab's name and sealed them with his seal, and sent letters to the elders and to the nobles who were living with Naboth in his city.

Now she wrote in the letters, saying, "Proclaim a fast and seat Naboth at the head of the people; and seat two worthless men before him, and let them testify against him, saying, 'You cursed God and the king.' Then take him out and stone him to death." So the men of his city, the elders and the nobles who lived in his city, did as Jezebel had sent word to them, just as it was written in the letters, which she had sent them. They proclaimed a fast and seated Naboth at the head of the people. Then the two worthless men came in and sat before him; and the worthless men testified against him, even against Naboth, before the people, saying, "Naboth cursed God and the king." So they took him outside the city and stoned him to death with stones.

---1 Kings 21:8–13

What did Jezebel proclaim?

What was her plan?

Jezebel proclaimed a *"false"* corporate fast to unjustly accuse Naboth and have him killed. Now, I'm sure this is not the type of fast God is seeking after. Jezebel also misused the law against Naboth. In Exodus 22:28, it says, "You shall not curse God, nor curse a ruler of your people. In Deuteronomy 19:15, it says, "A single witness shall not rise up against a man on account of any iniquity or any sin which he has committed; on the evidence of two or three witnesses a matter shall be confirmed. Therefore based on the misuse of the law and the lies of two worthless men, Naboth was martyred for standing for truth.

In Isaiah 58:3–4, the children of Israel were wondering why they could not get God's attention, despite them fasting and humbling themselves before God, they said: 'Why have we fasted and You do not see? Why have we humbled ourselves and You do not notice?' God answers them, behold, on the day of your fast you find your desire, and drive hard all your workers. "Behold, you fast for contention and strife and to strike with a wicked fist. You do not fast like you do today to make your voice heard on high.

WORD STUDY

The Hebrew word for **contention** is riybah, meaning: a strife, a controversy, a contention. The primary idea of this noun is that of a quarrel or dispute. It can be used in a legal sense to refer to an argument or case made in one's defense.

The Hebrew word for **strife** is matstsah, it refers to wrangling, quarreling and contention, especially brought on by arrogant or insolent attitudes, transgressions, and trespasses. It refers to the results of false fasts that brought on fighting, quarreling, and violence.

Ahab's sulking and not eating and Jezebels proclamation

of a fast in order to falsely accuse Naboth and incur violence upon him are both examples of false fasts. Israel pushing back their plates, yet making the work harder for those who worked for them and striking with a wicked fist is not the type of fast God desires.

When you are fasting, be aware of your actions and your reasons for fasting. If you are just going through the motions and don't have a humbled heart and not seeking God your fasting will be futile. It will be to no avail, you may loose a few pounds and gain some physical benefits but you will not have any spiritual gains.

CHAPTER 7

Ahab- An Idol Worshiper Gets God's Attention

Let's take another look at Ahab's character before we continue with the story in 1 Kings 21.

He was:

- King of Israel
- Walked in the sins of Jeroboam, the previous king *(for more information see 1Kings 14:7-11)*
- Married Jezebel

- Served and worshiped Baal, built an alter for Baal (idol worshiper)

- Made Asherah, which is a wooden symbol of a female deity

- He did more to provoke the Lord than all the kings before him

Picking back up with the story in the previous chapter, after Jezebel had Naboth stoned to death for refusing to sale his inherited land to Ahab, she shared the news with her husband and tells him to go and take possession of the land. Underline the message given to Ahab, by Elijah, in the passage below.

When Ahab heard that Naboth was dead, Ahab arose to go down to the vineyard of Naboth the Jezreelite, to take possession of it. Then the word of the LORD came to Elijah the Tishbite, saying, "Arise, go down to meet Ahab king of Israel, who is in Samaria; behold, he is in the vineyard of Naboth where he has gone down to take possession of it. "You shall speak to him, saying, 'Thus says the LORD, "Have you murdered and also taken possession?" ' And you shall speak to him, saying, 'Thus says the LORD, "In the place where the dogs licked up the blood of Naboth the dogs will lick up your blood, even yours." Ahab said to Elijah, "Have you found me, O my enemy?" And he answered, "I have found you, because you have sold yourself to do evil in the sight of the LORD. "Behold, I will bring evil upon you, and will utterly sweep you away, and will cut off from Ahab every male, both bond and free in Israel; and I will make your house like the house of Jeroboam the son of Nebat, and like the house of Baasha the son of Ahijah, because of the provocation with which you have provoked Me to anger, and because you have made Israel sin. "Of Jezebel also has the LORD spoken, saying, 'The dogs will eat Jezebel in the district of Jezreel.' "The one belonging to Ahab, who dies in the city, the dogs will eat, and the one who dies in the field the birds of heaven will eat." Surely there was no one like Ahab who sold himself to do evil in the sight of the LORD, because Jezebel his wife incited him. He acted very abominably in following idols, according to all that the Amorites had done, whom the LORD cast out before the sons of Israel.

---1 Kings 21:16–26

Who met Ahab in the vineyard?

What did Elijah say he had sold himself to do?

What message did Elijah have for Ahab?

What will happen to Ahab?

What will happen to his offspring?

What will happen to Jezebel?

What did Ahab make Israel do?

How is Ahab described?

Ahab is the king of Israel; he is supposed to be leading the people in the way of God the creator. Yet, he has decided to worship Baal, an idol, and not God. He has decided to marry a woman that doesn't worship the God of Israel. God is very angry with Ahab and Jezebel. They thought they would get away with murdering Naboth because of their position of power. They failed to realize that God is the ultimate ruler and there are consequences for breaking His laws.

Let's take a look at Ahab's response:

It came about when Ahab heard these words that

he tore his clothes and put on sackcloth and **fasted**, and he lay in sackcloth and went about despondently.

Then the word of the LORD came to Elijah the Tishbite, saying, "Do you see how Ahab has **humbled** himself before Me? Because he has **humbled** himself before Me, I will not bring the evil in his days, but I will bring the evil upon his house in his son's days."

---1 Kings 21:27–29

When Elijah delivered the message of the Lord to Ahab, Ahab humbled himself under the mighty hand of God. He tore his cloths, fasted, and lay in sackcloth and went about despondently. This got Gods attention! The man who worshipped idols, married a heathen, caused a nation to sin, and had a man killed because he wanted to plant a vegetable garden in his field, humbled himself, fasted and God responded.

This is a cause to rejoice! There is nothing you can do that can cause God to stop loving you. There is nothing that can separate you from his love. No matter how far you get off the path that he has set for you, there is a way

back.   And God is willing and ready to accept your
repentant heart.

CHAPTER 8

David- Repentance/Forgiveness

Many of you know the story of David and Bathsheba, found in 2 Samuel 11. Let's take a quick look at what happened. It was spring, the time the kings went to battle. This spring was different; David decided to stay in Jerusalem. One evening, he rolled out of bed and went for a walk on his roof. As he was walking on the roof, he saw a beautiful women bathing. David inquired about her, he found out her name was Bathsheba, she was the daughter of Eliam and she was married to Uriah. The fact that she was married didn't make a difference to David. He sent for her and lay with her. She reported to him that she was pregnant. David tried to cover it up by, sending for her husband who was on the battlefield. Uriah came home, but would not go to his house and lay with his wife. He didn't feel it would be right to eat, drink and lie with his wife while his comrades were on the battlefield. This was not going according to David's plan. He then comes up with a back up plan. He sends Uriah back to the battlefield with a letter. The letter stated that Uriah should be placed on the front line in the battle. Uriah was killed. David brought Bathsheba into his house and married her. God was not pleased with David's actions. In the following scriptures, underline all references to the rich man; circle all references to the poor man. Put a square around Nathan's response.

> Then the LORD sent Nathan *(the prophet)* to David. And he came to him and said, "There were two men in one city, the one rich and the other poor. "The rich man had a great many flocks and herds. "But the poor man had nothing except one little ewe lamb, which he bought and nourished; and it grew up together with him and his children. It would eat of his bread and drink of his cup and lie

in his bosom, and was like a daughter to him. "Now a traveler came to the rich man, and he was unwilling to take from his own flock or his own herd, to prepare for the wayfarer who had come to him; rather he took the poor man's ewe lamb and prepared it for the man who had come to him." Then David's anger burned greatly against the man, and he said to Nathan, "As the LORD lives, surely the man who has done this deserves to die. "He must make restitution for the lamb fourfold, because he did this thing and had no compassion." Nathan then said to David, "You are the man! Thus says the LORD God of Israel, 'It is I who anointed you king over Israel and it is I who delivered you from the hand of Saul.

---2 Samuel 12:1–7

What did you learn about the rich man?

What did you learn about the poor man?

What did David say the rich man's punishment should be?

What was Nathan's response?

David's response:

> Then David said to Nathan, "I have sinned against the LORD." And Nathan said to David, "The LORD also has taken away your sin; you shall not die. "However, because by this deed you have given occasion to the enemies of the LORD to blaspheme,

the child also that is born to you shall surely die."

---2 Samuel 12:13–14

David realized that he had sinned against the Lord. He also knew that under the Levitical law, he and Bathsheba were both suppose to be put to death. Leviticus 20:10 says, 'If there is a man who commits adultery with another man's wife, one who commits adultery with his friend's wife, the adulterer and the adulteress shall surely be put to death.' Instead of death, David receives grace. This is a foreshadow of Christ's redemptive power, David's sins are taken away. Yet, there were still consequences for his sin. In the following passage underline the consequences of David's rebellion against God.

'Why have you despised the word of the LORD by doing evil in His sight? You have struck down Uriah the Hittite with the sword, have taken his wife to be your wife, and have killed him with the sword of the sons of Ammon. 'Now therefore, the sword shall never depart from your house, because you have despised Me and have taken the wife of Uriah the Hittite to be your wife.'

"Thus says the LORD, 'Behold, I will raise up evil against you from your own household; I will even take your wives before your eyes and give *them* to your companion, and he will lie with your wives in broad daylight. 'Indeed you did it secretly, but I will do this thing before all Israel, and under the sun.' " "However, because by this deed you have given occasion to the enemies of the LORD to blaspheme, the child also that is born to you shall surely die."

---2 Samuel 12:9–12, 14

WORD STUDY

Despised-definition: careless, contempt, despicable, disdained

Now, list the consequences David faced for despising the

word of the Lord.

Let's take a look at what David did next:

> David therefore inquired of God for the child; and David fasted and went and lay all night on the ground. The elders of his household stood beside him in order to raise him up from the ground, but he was unwilling and would not eat food with them. Then it happened on the seventh day that the child died. And the servants of David were afraid to tell him that the child was dead, for they said, "Behold, while the child was still alive, we spoke to him and he did not listen to our voice. How then can we tell him that the child is dead, since he might do himself harm!"
>
> But when David saw that his servants were whispering together, David perceived that the child was dead; so David said to his servants, "Is the child dead?" And they said, "He is dead."

> ---2 Samuel 12:16–19

How does David respond?

So David arose from the ground, washed, anointed himself, and changed his clothes; and he came into the house of the LORD and worshiped. Then he came to his own house, and when he requested, they set food before him and he ate.

---2 Samuel 12:20

List David's actions in verse 20:

In the midst of this very painful situation David recognized the sovereignty of God over life and death. God chose to take David's son home. David responded by washing, anointing himself, putting on a fresh set of cloths and entering into the house of the Lord to worship Him.

In the following verses underline David's response.

Then his servants said to him, "What is this thing that you have done? While the child was alive, you fasted and wept; but when the child died, you arose and ate food." He (David) said, "While the child was still alive, I fasted and wept; for I said, 'Who knows, the LORD may be gracious to me, that the child may live.' "But now he has died; why should I fast? Can I bring him back again? I will go to him, but he will not return to me."

---2 Samuel 12:21–23

We can learn a lot from David. When a loved one is sick we find ourselves covering them in prayer. Petitioning God for His healing power to rest upon them. Many times He hears and answer by restoring them back to health. Other times He heals by taking them home. Whatever God decides to do, our response should be like David's; we should worship God, especially when a believer goes home to be with the Lord. In addition to worshipping God we should live out the rest of our days fulfilling God's plan and purpose in our lives. So that when our days are complete we can hear him say well done my good and faithful servant.

Next it says:

Then David comforted his wife Bathsheba, and

went in to her and lay with her; and she gave birth to a son, and he named him Solomon. Now the LORD loved him.

----2 Samuel 12:24

David recognized that in all that he had done, ultimately he had sinned against God. He responded by **humbling** himself, **praying, fasting** and **surrendering to God's will**. This got God's attention. God didn't relent on His word; yet, David and Bathsheba were blessed with the birth of a baby boy, Solomon.

The book of Psalms, gives us some insight on how David felt when Nathan came to him and pointed out his sin, "you are the man", 2 Samuel 12:7.

Take your time as you go through Psalm 51

Be gracious to me, O God, according to Your lovingkindness; According to the greatness of Your compassion blot out my **transgressions**. Wash me thoroughly from my **iniquity** and cleanse me from my **sin**. For I know my **transgressions**, and my **sin** is ever before me. Against You, You only, I have sinned and done what is evil in Your sight, So that You are justified when You speak And blameless when You judge.

----Psalm 51:1–4

WORD STUDY

Transgressions (Pesha)- willful deviation from the path of righteousness, premeditated crossing of the line of God's law, a rebellious act of rejecting God's authority, a revolt

Iniquity (Awon)- a depraved action, perversity, denotes deeds and consequences, results in separation from God, alienation and uncleanness. Man must be aware of Awon and confess it, change his way of life. God will forgive

Sin (chattath)-youthful discretions, an offense, to miss the mark

What does David ask God to do?

How does David describe sin?

Who did David sin against?

Continuing with Psalm 51:

> Behold, I was brought forth in iniquity, and in sin my mother conceived me.
>
> Behold, You desire truth in the innermost being, and in the hidden part You will make me know wisdom. Purify me with hyssop, and I shall be clean; Wash me, and I shall be whiter than snow. Make me to hear joy and gladness,

let the bones which You have broken rejoice. Hide Your face from my sins and blot out all my iniquities.

----Psalm 51:5–9

What does God desire?

What does David ask God to do?

In the following verses underline David's request.

Create in me a clean heart, O God, And renew a steadfast spirit within me.

Do not cast me away from Your presence And do not take Your Holy Spirit from me. Restore to me the joy of Your salvation and sustain me with a willing spirit. Then I will teach transgressors Your ways, and sinners will be converted to You.

--- Psalm 51: 10-13

What does David ask God to do?

What will David Do?

In the passage below, circle the type of sacrifice that God wants.

Deliver me from bloodguiltiness, O God, the God of my salvation; then my tongue will joyfully sing of Your righteousness. O Lord, open my lips, that my mouth may declare Your praise. For You do not delight in sacrifice, otherwise I would give it; You are not pleased with burnt offering. The sacrifices of God are a broken spirit; a broken and a contrite heart, O God, You will not despise.

---Psalm 51:14–17

David humbled himself under the mighty hand of God. He new he had messed up. He was aware that when he sinned he had sinned against God. He asks God to blot out his transgressions and iniquities, create within him a new heart and a steadfast spirit. When we have sinned against God we should follow this example. Humble ourselves, acknowledge our sin and ask God for forgiveness. We shouldn't be condemned by our sin and find ourselves far from God. He wants us to bring our broken spirit and heart to Him. This He will not despise. This will get God's attention.

Psalm 32, is a Psalm written around the same time as Psalm 51. This Psalm gives us more insight into how David responded, after he was confronted by the Lord, through Nathan. Read the passage below and underline each occurrence of the word blessed.

How blessed is he whose transgression is forgiven, whose sin is covered! How blessed is the man to whom the LORD does not impute iniquity and in whose spirit there is no deceit! When I kept silent about my sin, my body wasted away through my groaning all day long. For day and night your hand was heavy upon me; my vitality was drained away as with the fever heat of summer.

----Psalm 32:1-4

What do you learn about those who are blessed?

What happened to David when he was silent about his sin?

God forgives sin. He sent His son, Jesus Christ to die for the sins of the world. When we ask God for forgiveness, He forgives. When David didn't acknowledge his sin, it manifested as a physical illness.

In the following scripture, underline all references to Lord and any synonyms -Thee, Thou, You, etc.

I acknowledged my sin to Thee and my iniquity I did not hide; I said, "I will confess my transgressions to the Lord"; And You forgave the guilt of my sin. Therefore, let everyone who is godly pray to Thee in a time when You may be found; Surely in a flood of great waters they will not reach him. Thou art my hiding place; Thou dost preserve me from trouble; Thou dost surround me with songs of deliverance.

----Psalm 32:5-7

What did you learn about the Lord in this passage?

What did the Lord forgive?

WORD STUDY

Guilt- definition: iniquity, the guilt that results from the act of sin

This is so freeing, not only does God forgive our sin, He also forgives the guilt that results from the act of the sin. Since God is a forgiving God and doesn't remember our sins, why do we hold on to sin? We have a tendency to rehearse our past, not letting it go. God says he has cast them into the sea of forgetfulness, yet we replay it over and over again in our minds. We live with regret; we live in shame because of past actions. Yet, God has redeemed us, He has set us free. Let it go, walk in the freedom that God has made available for you today.

Let's take a look at another Psalm. Psalm 18 is written in parallel to 2 Samuel 22, after David was delivered from the hand of all his enemies, including his son Absalom and Saul.   Underline the words Lord, God and all synonyms. Make a list of what you learn about the LORD in this passage. Reread the passage and circle words referring to David, such as I, my, me. Record David's response.

"I love You, O LORD, my strength." The LORD is my rock and my fortress and my deliverer, My God, my rock, in whom I take refuge; My shield and the horn of my salvation, my stronghold. I call upon the LORD, who is worthy to be praised, And I am saved from my enemies. The cords of death encompassed me, And the torrents of ungodliness terrified me. The cords of Sheol surrounded me; The snares of death confronted me. In my distress I called upon the LORD, And cried to my God for help; He heard my voice out of His temple, And my cry for help before Him came into His ears

----Psalm 18:1–6

LORD:

David:

Continue marking references to Lord and David in the passage below. Take notice of how David views himself after he sins against God.

He sent from on high, He took me; He drew me out of many waters. He delivered me from my strong enemy, And from those who hated me, for they were too mighty for me. They confronted me in the day of my calamity, but the LORD was my stay. He brought me forth also into a broad place; He rescued me, because He delighted in me. The LORD has rewarded me according to my righteousness; According to the cleanness of my hands He has recompensed me. For I have kept the ways of the LORD, and have not wickedly departed from my God. For all His ordinances were before me, and I did not put away His statutes from me. I was also blameless with Him, and I kept myself from my iniquity. Therefore the LORD has recompensed me according to my righteousness, According to the cleanness of my hands in His eyes.

----Psalm 18:16–24

What did you learn from marking LORD and its synonyms?

How does David describe himself?

How dos God view David?

Does David accept God's forgiveness?

When we sin, we sin against God. When we ask for forgiveness, we should believe that God has forgiven us and walk in that forgiveness. We should not hold on to the things of the past. Philippians 3:13-14 says, brethren, I do not regard myself as having laid hold of it yet; but one thing I do: forgetting what lies behind and reaching forward to what lies ahead, I press on toward the goal for the prize of the upward call of God in Christ Jesus. Paul says, we should forget what lies behind and reach forward to what lies ahead. God's word also says that He has taken our sins from us, as far as the east is from the west. Therefore, we should walk in this freedom of forgiveness that has been made available to us, and press toward the goal that God has set before us. No matter what we may have done, we should see ourselves as David saw himself; righteous, clean, blameless in the eyes of our Lord and Savior.

Part 2

A Guide To Healthy Fasting

CHAPTER 9

Physical Benefits Of Fasting

We've looked at many examples of how to get God's attention in fasting. Now I would like to shift gears a little and take a look at how fasting affects the physical body. In a biblical fast, we get the benefit of getting Gods attention through prayer, humility, repentance, and seeking His face. Please don't take out the time to abstain from food, making a physical sacrifice without getting the spiritual rewards. ...He is a rewarder of those who diligently seek Him, Hebrews 11:6. Seek Him intentionally, expect Him to respond, look for the rewards.

Before we can look at the physical we must go back to the beginning. When God spoke this world into existence.

In the beginning God created the heavens and the earth. The earth was formless and void, and darkness was over the surface of the deep, and the Spirit of God was moving over the surface of the waters. Then God said, "Let there be light"; and there was light. God saw that the light was good; and God separated the light from the darkness. God called the light day, and the darkness He called night. And there was evening and there was morning, one day.

----Gen 1: 1-5

Genesis 1:1 says " in the beginning God created the heavens and the earth". Let's take a look at His creation and see how it relates to us today. But before we do that let's look at the definition of created. In Hebrew the word for created is *Bārā* it means to create, form, make, produce, bring into existence. Bārā emphasizes the initiation of the object, not manipulating it after original creation. It refers only to an activity, which can be performed by God. Therefore; In the beginning God created, formed, produced, brought into existence the heavens and the earth from nothing.

> All things came into being through Him, and apart from Him nothing came into being that has come into being.
>
> ---- John 1:3

> The earth was formless and void, and darkness was over the surface of the deep, and the Spirit of God was moving over the surface of the waters
>
> ---Genesis 1:2

In Genesis 1:2, the earth was described as formless, void, and dark but the Spirit of

God was present. He moved over the surface of the waters. The analogy of "moved over the surface of the water" is like a fowl continually brooding over hatching eggs. God had a plan and purpose for earth and when God is present, things just can't remain the same.

Then God said, "Let there be light"; and there was light. God saw that the light was good; and God separated the light from the darkness. God called the light day, and the darkness He called night. And there was evening and there was morning, one day.

----Genesis 1:3-5

When God spoke there was an immediate result. When He said, "let there be light," at His command light appeared. He saw that the light was good and separated light from darkness. Day and night were established. Many times when we think about night and day, we think about the sun creating light and night is when the sun goes down and the moon rises. Yet at this particular time, in the process of creation, the sun and moon have yet to be created. On the first day of creation there is a separation of light and darkness. I find it interesting that separation of light and darkness is one of the first recorded actions taken by God. We see Him still performing this action today with his people, for example:

> For you are all sons of light and sons of day. We are not of night nor of darkness.

> ----1 Thessalonians 5:5

> I have come as Light into the world, so that everyone who believes in Me will not remain in darkness.

> ---- John 12:46

> You are the light of the world. A city set on a hill cannot be hidden; nor does anyone light a lamp and put it under a basket, but on the lampstand, and it gives light to all who are in the house. Let your light shine before men in such a way that they may see your good works, and

glorify your Father who is in heaven.

----Matthew 5:14-16

You may be asking how is this relevant to my health? One example of the relevance of day and night is, scientist found small nuclei in the hypothalamus of the brain called the suprachiasmatic nucleus (SCN). These nuclei are responsible for controlling circadian rhythms of all living organisms; bacteria, plants, fungi, animals, and humans. Franz Halberg introduced the concept of the circadian rhythm in 1959. The circadian rhythm was found to function in a 24-hour cycle and respond to light and darkness. The circadian rhythm influences the sleep wake cycle, body temperature, hormone secretion, cell division and proliferation, gastro-intestinal tract function, reproductive function, metabolism, and body mass regulation. Let's take a deeper look into how the circadian rhythm affects the gastro-intestinal tract. God has designed our bodies, to process food and nutrients at a higher capacity during the day. More energy is geared toward the intestine during the daytime, than during the night. Insulin secretion is more abundant during the day, as compared to night. In other words, our bodies are equipped to take in food, break it down, absorb nutrients and discard waste, and produce energy, better in the day than during the night. The gastro-intestinal tract was formed to rest during the night. Advancements in lighting, technology, etc. have changed the way man operates in a 24-hour day. In the days of Adam and Eve, when the sun went down, most activity ceased. Food was eaten during the day, when it was available. Portions of these resources were stored for utilization during the rest of the day and night, the fasting period, without compromising fitness and vitality. Today, it is convenient to go to the kitchen and whip up a late night snack, and then go to bed. This compromises the fasting period that our bodies were designed to have.

Another practical example is how the circadian rhythm affects the absorption of sugar. God designed the cells to be more sensitive to processing carbohydrates and sugar during the day than in the evening. For example, the cells are better able to absorb the glucose from a glass of fresh orange juice in the daytime, than in the evening. For those dealing with blood sugar issues, this is a great clinical pearl. As a rule of thumb, you want to limit your sugar and carbohydrate intake. It is better to consume these foods in the earlier part of the day than in the afternoon or evening. I believe one of the reasons why we are seeing an increase in metabolic disease is not only due to the overconsumption of sugar and carbohydrates, but it is also related to the time that we consume these products.

I have my patients commit to a 8-10 hour window of when they will eat. They only have water or unsweetened herbal tea outside of this window. In my practice, I have seen this step alone help transform lives. Patients have reported better self control over what they eat, increased energy, better sleep, less gas and bloating, and better blood sugar regulation. Getting back to the basics, the way God intended for us to eat, can make a difference.

When fasting is incorporated with the 8-10 hour window, this only enhances the bodies ability to perform at its highest level. Just think about it, if you eat three meals a day, 365 days a year, (not *including* snacks), that amounts to 1,095 meals per year. The body has to digest the food, extract the nutrients, and discard the waste. So giving the body a break with a fast for a 1 day, 3 day, 21 day, 28 day or 40 day fast will give the body much needed rest. When the body is given time to rest and detox, we begin to see healing occur.

Physical Rewards Associated With Fasting:

- Increased Immunity
- Hard coating of mucus on the intestinal wall removed
- Cleansing of the lymphatic system and bloodstream

- Toxins removed from the spleen, liver, and kidneys
- Mucus from the lungs and sinuses will be removed, breathing becomes fuller, freer and deeper
- Excess cholesterol broken down and removed from the body
- Rapid, safe weight loss is achieved without flabbiness
- Organs are revitalized
- The skin becomes silky, soft, and sensitive
- There is greater ease of movement-arthritic joints will feel much better
- Increased Energy
- Weight loss- burn fat
- Inflammation reduced
- Intestines get a break- healing occurs
- Glucose levels reduced
- Blood pressure reduced
- Insulin sensitivity improved
- Decreased risk for chronic disease
- Better sleep
- Improved mental clarity
- Stem cell activity increased
- Cellular Autophagy stimulated

- White blood cells increase
- Decrease risk of breast cancer and reoccurrence
- Decrease side effects to chemotherapy

CHAPTER 10

What The Research Says About Fasting

Research is finally identifying what God promised thousands of years ago, through His prophet, Isaiah. As we take a look at Isaiah 58, we see that when we fast...*your recovery will speedily spring forth* in verse 8 and that God will *give strength to your bones* in verse 11. We can finally see the evidence of this actually occurring in the body.

Is not this the fast that I have chosen: to loose the bonds of wickedness, to undo the bands of the yoke, and to let the oppressed go free, and that ye break every yoke? Is it not to deal thy bread to the hungry, and that thou bring the poor that are cast out to thy house? when thou seest the naked, that thou cover him; and that thou hide not thyself from thine own flesh? Then shall thy light break forth as the morning, and thy healing shall spring forth speedily; and thy righteousness shall go before thee; the glory of Jehovah shall be thy rear guard. Then shalt thou call, and Jehovah will answer; thou shalt cry, and he will say, Here I am...and Jehovah will guide thee continually, and satisfy thy soul in dry places, and make strong thy bones; and thou shalt be like a watered garden, and like a spring of water, whose waters fail not.

----Isaiah 58:6-11

Lets' take a look at a few studies:

A recent study showed that fasting for a minimum of three days can regenerate the entire immune system. Researchers have found this to be very beneficial for the elderly and for cancer patients. As we age, our immune system becomes weaker and it becomes harder to fight infections. Fasting causes the **bone** marrow to produce new white blood cells (...***giving strength to your bones***). White blood cells are our bodies defense system. Their job is to recognize bacteria, viruses, and cancer cells and rid the body of these foreign invaders. When damaged white blood cells are broken down during fasting this encourages the body to create new undamaged white blood cells; therefore regenerating a whole new immune system. These new white blood cells are not damaged therefore can recognize foreign invaders and cancer and rid them from the body (***...your recovery will speedily spring forth).***

Research also showed that fasting for 72 hours protected patients against the toxic effects of chemotherapy.

A study by JAMA Oncology was published on the affects of fasting and a recurrence of breast cancer. The findings were very encouraging. The researchers collected data from 2,413 women who had previously had breast cancer. They were between the ages of 27 to 70 years old when they were diagnosed with breast cancer. They all participated in the prospective Women's Healthy Eating and Living study between 1995 and 2007. The data was analyzed to measure the outcome of breast cancer recurrence and new primary tumors forming for a period of 7.3 years and death from breast cancer or any cause for 11.4 years. The results showed that participants who broke their fast, had less than 13 hours between their evening and morning meals, had a 36% higher chance of breast cancer recurrence compared with those who fasted 13 or more hours, nightly. They also found that longer nightly fasting reduced HbA_{1C} levels. This is encouraging because as a naturopathic doctor I am always looking for non-invasive, natural ways to prevent disease from occurring. And based on these findings, just by simply extending the length of nightly fasting could be a medication free strategy to reduce the return of breast cancer and help reverse diabetes.

Another study, researching patients with Type 2 diabetes was done to see if fasting had any beneficial effects. The study included 46 patients. They restricted their food intake to 300kcal/day for 7 days in the form of liquids only. The benefits found were: weight loss, reductions of weight in the abdominal area, a decrease in blood pressure, systolic as well as diastolic blood pressure, increased quality of life and improvement in insulin and Hemoglobin A1c levels.

Researchers have also studied different types of fast, such as intermittent fasting, modified fasting, time restricted diets, and calorie restricted fasts. Below is an overview of these fasts and there benefits.

Intermittent Fasting-intermittent fasting is regularly allowing greater than normal amounts of time to pass between meals. A few examples are skipping breakfast or dinner, fasting every 3 days, one day a week, or once a month. Research shows that intermittent fasting can decrease your risk of cancer, cancer reoccurrence, cardiovascular disease, type II diabetes, and obesity. It can protect against Alzheimer's and Parkinson's disease, improve memory, sleep, energy, and have an overall feeling of well-being. A study that consisted of males showed that intermittent fasting decreased tension, anger, and confusion. Another study stated that intermittent fasting may contribute to the prevention and treatment of chronic diseases *(... your recovery will speedily spring forth)*.

Modified fasting- modified fasting regimens generally refer to limiting energy, food, consumption. Modified fasting limits food to 20–25% of energy needs on regularly scheduled fasting days. This type of regimen, also called intermittent energy restriction. This is the basis for the popular 5:2 diet, which involves energy, food, restriction for 2 nonconsecutive days per week and unrestricted eating during the other 5 days of the week. For example, only eating one meal on Mondays and

Wednesday's, and 3 meals a day, on Tuesday, Thursday, Friday, Saturday, and Sunday. Nine studies were reviewed, the studies ranged from 2 to 6 months. Of the nine studies, only one included weekly exercise goals. Overall, the results reported statistically significant weight loss, which ranged from 3.2% in comparison to 8.0%. There was also a significant decrease in fasting insulin, and fasting glucose. There were improvements in LDL cholesterol, triglycerides, improvements in inflammatory markers, including C-reactive protein, tumor necrosis factor-α, adiponectin, leptin, and brain-derived neurotrophic factor. The participants also reported improvements in mood, including reductions in anger, tension, and fatigue. They reported an increase in self-confidence and positive mood. There were a few negative side effects, such as feeling cold, irritable, low energy, or hunger.

Time Restricted Diet- Time-restricted feeding (TRF) is a daily eating pattern in which all nutrient intake occurs within a few hours (usually ≤12h) everyday, with no overt attempt to alter nutrient quality or quantity. The concept of TRF arose within the context of circadian rhythms. Circadian rhythms are daily ~24h rhythms in metabolism, physiology and behavior that are sustained under constant light or dark conditions. An example is the 16:8 diet, fasting for 16 hours and eating within an 8 hour window. Studies showed that when patients restrict food to a 8-10 hour window, there was a decrease in weight, blood pressure, blood sugar levels, insulin sensitivity, chronic diseases, and oxidative stress.

Calorie Restricted Fast- According to the research, restricting calories between 400-600 calories per day, will allow you to reap the healing benefits from fasting. There are many ways to restrict calorie consumption. For example, drinking water only, herbal tea, fresh vegetable juice, or bone broth, or fasting mimicking diets.

Beloved, I pray that in all things thou mayest prosper and be in health, even as thy soul prospereth

--
3John2

CHAPTER 11

Fasting As A Lifestyle

To reap the physical benefits of fasting, incorporating fasting on a regular basis would be very beneficial. There are many options for fasting, according to the research, that have restorative benefits:

- 24 hour fast-once a week, water or herbal tea only. Example from dinner to dinner, or lunch to lunch

- 2 days a week-eating 5 days a week and restricting food intake 2 nonconsecutive days a week.

- Daily fasting- 8-10 hour window-for example, 8 hour feeding period, followed by 16-hour fasting period. Eating between 8am-4pm, only drinking water or unsweetened herbal tea outside this window.

- Extended fasts, 3 days or longer

- Calorie restriction fasts- 400-500 calories

Personally, I incorporate intermittent fasting on a daily basis, only eating within an 8-10-hour window. During the month of February, I participate in a 28-29 day extended corporate fast/prayer with Sound Words Christian Education and All Nations Church, that incorporates only liquids. Periodically, during the year, I restrict food intake, humble myself, and seek His face. Incorporating fasting, as a lifestyle will allow you to reap the spiritual and physical benefits of fasting.

When you fast, remove solid food from your diet, your body will begin to breakdown toxins, harmful substances accumulating in the body. Incorporating fresh juices, and herbal teas, that are full of antioxidants, will help the detoxing process by binding to toxins and help rid them from the body. Vegetables are considered as "builders", they help rebuild the immune system and aid in repair while fruits are "cleansers", they aide in cleansing the body. A word of caution, when using fresh juices during a fast, do not make the mistake in drinking copious amounts of fruit juice. An abundance of fruit juice will elevate your blood sugar levels. You will find yourself feeling good, very energetic and then your body crashes, due to an elevated blood sugar level that crashes suddenly. The goal is to keep blood sugar levels steady. Concentrating on water, herbal tea, vegetable juice and broth will have more of a stabilizing affect on blood sugar levels.

What is occurring during an extended fast (3 days or longer)?

Three phases of fasting:

Phase 1- six hours after your last meal the body uses glucose, amino acids and fat to fuel the body

Phase 2- two days after your last meal, the body begins to use glucose stores called glycogen. This is stored glucose found in the liver and muscle cells.

Phase 3- approximately three days after your last meal, the body begins to convert fat into fuel, ketosis. This is when weight loss begins. Stem cells are stimulated, there is an increase in autophagy, (cleaning up cellular debris), and human growth hormone.

After Phase 3- Hunger and cravings reduced significantly

During phase two and three you may become irritable, more emotional than usual, have hunger pangs, require more sleep, experience headaches, have a white coat on your tongue, and have bad breath. Don't be alarmed; these are signs that your body is detoxifying. A great way to relieve these symptoms is by sweating and doing a coffee enema. Instructions found in appendix.

When your metabolism slows down due to a decrease in caloric intake your body temperature will drop and you will be colder than normal. If fasting during the winter months be sure to drink plenty of warm liquids, you may also add cayenne pepper to your liquids. Sitting in an infrared sauna will help warm you up and aid in removing toxins from your body. It is important that you sweat, during a fast. You want to mobilize toxins from fat cells and out of the body through sweating. This can be done several ways: Hot bath while drinking herbal tea, sitting in a sauna, or exercising.

If you begin to experience back pain this may be an indication that you are dehydrated. Remember to drink at least half your body weight in ounces daily. It is a good idea to get in the habit of drinking 1-2 cups of water within 15 minutes upon waking. Staying well hydrated will decrease hunger pains and keep your bowels moving appropriately. This will also help you remove toxins from your body.

If you become constipated, make sure you are drinking at least ½ your body weight in ounces daily. Apply castor oil packs over the abdomen three to four times a week. Drinking Smooth move herbal tea, or aloe vera juice may help stimulate bowel motility. Magnesium 500mg, also helps stimulate the bowel. Consider doing several enemas and/or colonics while on an extended fast.

Don't give up. These symptoms won't last long, usually only a few days. Joy is coming in the morning!

... weeping may endure for a night, but joy cometh in the morning

---Psalm30:5

CHAPTER 12

Common Questions Asked About Fasting:

Should I exercise while fasting?

Yes, exercise is very beneficial. It aids in the cleansing process. It helps your body release toxins. You may not be able to exercise as much as you did prior to fasting, listen to your body. When you are feeling tired stop, or only do light exercises. The days you are feeling energetic, you can increase your regime. If you didn't exercise regularly, prior to fasting, walking 30 minutes a day is a great place to start.

Should I take supplements?

When I first started doing extended fasts, I recommended not taking supplements during this time. But due to expanded knowledge, I have changed my position in this area. Certain nutrients are necessary to mobilize toxins stored in tissue to be removed from the body. The liver requires vitamins and minerals for detoxification. Therefore, I recommend taking one whole food vitamin daily and Magnesium. I also like to replenish good bacteria, probiotics, to establish bowel health. Heavy metals, insecticides, pesticides, and minerals are lost when we sweat; therefore after working out or sauna use, it would be good to take a mineral supplement to replace lost minerals.

I feel tired should I push myself and do what needs to be done?

It is important to listen to your body. Some days you

will require more rest, take the time rest. Restoration and repair are occurring on a cellular level. Make sure you are well hydrated, drinking ½ your body weight in ounces of liquid daily.

How do I handle the hunger pains?

In my experience, it is easy to get caught up in daily tasks and not drink enough water. It is important that you are well hydrated. You should consume at least ½ your body weight in ounces of liquid daily. If your lips or mouth becomes dry, you need water. If you experience low back pain, you need water. While at work, I keep liquids on my desk, and when I am out running errands, I always take liquids with me. This helps me stay well hydrated throughout the day. Also limiting television helps with hunger pains by deceasing your exposure to ALL those commercials with tempting delicacies.

I just can't seem to get warm enough, what should I do?

During fasting, your body temperature will drop a

little. A few ways to keep warm, especially if your fasting during the winter months are to: Drink warm liquids-herbal tea, add cayenne pepper to water, ginger shots-juice 2oz of fresh ginger root, take warm baths while sipping on herbal tea, sit in the sauna.

I feel nauseated, what should I do?

Nausea while fasting may occur. This may be due to your body releasing toxins into the system too fast. One way to combat this issue is to decrease beet juice; beet juice tends to detox the liver quickly. Increase herbal tea that has liver supporting herbs such as milk thistle, chaparral, ginger root, and garlic. Sweat, sweating will aid your body in releasing toxins. Taking a whole food multivitamin can help supply your body with nutrients needed for detoxification. Some patients benefit from taking a scoop of rice/pea protein-Mediclear Plus. Mediclear Plus supplies the body with all the necessary nutrients for liver detoxification, eliminating nausea.

(Where to purchase supplements found in the Appendix)

What if I mess up and break the fast, should I just quite?

If you have a moment of weakness and break the fast, don't worry. Don't condemn yourself. God does not condemn you. He understands that the flesh is weak. Just jump right back on. Remember to seek God first, stay in your word and pray regularly. One exercise I do is, whenever I begin to feel hungry, I begin to pray. I use the hunger pains as a reminder to pray. Also prepare before the fast begins. Have a list of juices, broths, smoothie recipes prepared before your fast begins. This way you will not find yourself spending hours on the Internet searching for recipes during the fast.

CHAPTER 13

Breaking An Extended Fast Safely

Extended fasts are fasts that last three days or longer.

Turning on the digestive system can take one to seven days, depending on the length of the fast. So reintroduction of food into your digestive system is important. The key is to take it slow, listen to your body, watch your quantities and seek guidance from the Lord.

1. Digestion begins in the mouth. Saliva has enzymes that assist in digestion. The enzymes in saliva can digest up to 80 percent starch, 30 percent protein and 10 percent fat. Therefore eat slowly and chew food well. During the first week, break the fast with soft, juicy foods such as watermelon and cantaloupe. Cabbage and beets can be grated cabbage adding the juice of an orange or lemon for dressing. Eating slowly and chewing food well will gently awaken your digestive system. Do not break a fast by eating meat, bread, canned soups, or junk food. This can cause stomach cramps, nausea and weakness, negating much of the benefits of the fast.

2. During the second week gradually increase quantities and variety of food. Begin to incorporate carrots, onions, potatoes, celery, etc. into your diet. Dried fruit and nuts can also be added in the second week.

3. During the third week work on maintaining a healthy balanced diet. Eat raw and cooked vegetables, organic when possible. Continue to eat fruit and drink 1/2 your body weight in ounces of water daily. Add rice, quinoa, couscous, and whole-wheat pasta. Avoid dairy, deep fried foods, sugar, and artificial sweeteners.

4. Do not overeat! Discover the amount of food that your body needs to live a vibrant, healthy life.

5. Continue to pray. God should be just as much a part of your eating, as He was part of your fasting.

6. Educate yourself on how to begin a lifestyle of healthy eating. Fasting is a wonderful new beginning, a foundation for a lifelong, healthy diet. So that you can continue to reap the spiritual and physical rewards.

CHAPTER 14

RECIPES

Fresh juices

- 2-3 apples, 1/2 - 1 small beet, 1 inch ginger, 2-3 stalks celery
- 5 kale leaves, 2-3 apples, 1/2 lemon, 1 prune
- 5 carrots, 2 apples, 1 inch ginger
- Handful of berries, ½ lemon

This means you should get a juicer. A juicer is different from a blender, vitamix or nutri-bullet. A juicer removes the fiber from the vegetables and fruit. When fiber is removed the nutrients are able to go directly to cellular level. When vitamins, minerals and enzymes in the fresh juice go directly to the cells the digestive system is bypassed and the nutrients are used to fuel the cells. When cells are provided with the proper nutrients healing occurs.

When juicing, it is important to use more vegetables than fruit. Fruit juices have a tendency to raise blood sugar levels.

Homemade broth

Add vegetables and herbs- onion, garlic, carrots, beets with leaves, potatoes, curry, kale, spinach, celery, cayenne pepper to water, boil, strain, drink the broth.

Homemade broth is suggested because you determine what you put in the broth and the sodium content. High levels of sodium on a liquid fast may cause physical complications like headache and stomach cramps. Home made vegetable broth will provide you with nutrients and something to warm you up.

Infused Water

Add ingredients to water, let infuse minimum of 30 minutes up to a few hours

- 2 slices of lemon, and orange

- 2 strawberries, a few blueberries, 2 slices of lemon
- 2 slices of apple or peach, 2 slices of lemon, 1 cinnamon stick
- Lime slices- help regulate blood sugar

Use organic fruit-fruit free from insecticides and pesticides-. The goal is to limit toxin exposure, not to increase it.

APPENDIX

How To Make A Coffee Enema?

Coffee enema is simply an effective and natural process to cleanse our body. The liver is our primary processor of all the blood in the body. All the blood in the body passes through the liver every 3 minutes. Coffee enema cleanses the toxins and wastes in the blood by stimulating the liver to make more bile.

Coffee Enema Kits

1. Reusable enema kit
2. Organic coffee which is not decaffeinated
3. Pot for cooking coffee
4. Distilled water

Prepare a coffee enema

1. Mix 3 tablespoons of coffee to 1 quart of distilled water in a pot and boil it for 3 minutes and simmer for 15 minutes.
2. Strain and use at body temperature.

Coffee Enema Instructions

1. Pour 2cups into a reusable enema bag.
2. Hang it at a door knob or something that is almost the same height.
3. Open the clamp and release some coffee out to make sure no air is in the tube.
4. Add olive oil, or vitamin E to the end of the tube.

5. Lie down on the floor. You can put a mat or towel on the floor.

6. Insert tube into anus
7. Allow the coffee to start going in your body and hold it for 15 minutes.
8. Release the coffee into the toilet bowl

How often do you do a coffee enema?

If you are having some health problems, it is recommended to do coffee enema once a day. If you are someone who is very healthy, do it once a week. If you have constipation very often, do coffee enema 2 to 3 times per week.

Supplement Purchase:

Supplements can also be purchased in office at:
4421 Salem Ave
Dayton OH 45416

Websites:
www.DSSOrders.com/DrEdwards
Registration code: VE1366
Coupon code:HCPC1366WELCOME-20% discount on first order,
HCPC1366MEDICLEAR-20% discount on Mediclear Plus

https://wellevate.me/vanessa-edwards

NPscript.com practitioner passcode: Drvedwards

Bibliography

Edwards, Vanessa. *Fasting to Spiritual and Physical Health.* Vanessa Edwards, 2018.

Halberg, Nils, et al. "Effect of Intermittent Fasting and Refeeding on Insulin Action in Healthy Men." *Journal of Applied Physiology*, vol. 99, no. 6, 2005, pp. 2128–2136., doi:10.1152/japplphysiol.00683.2005.

Hussin NM, Shahar S, Teng NI, Ngah WZ, Das SK. 2013. *Efficacy of fasting and calorie restriction on mood and depression among ageing men.* Epub 2013

Knapton, Sarah. 2014. *Fasting for three days can regenerate entire immune system, study finds.* The Telegraph

Jockers, david. "Registration." *Fasting Transformation Summit*, 2018, fastingtransformation.com/.

Lankelma J, Kooi B, Krab K, Dorsman JC, Joenje H, Westerhoff HV. 2015. *A reason for intermittent fasting to suppress the awakening of dormant breast tumors.* Epub 2014 Nov 4

Li, Chenying, et al. "Effects of A One-Week Fasting Therapy in Patients with Type-2 Diabetes Mellitus and Metabolic Syndrome – A Randomized Controlled Explorative Study." *Experimental and Clinical Endocrinology & Diabetes*, vol. 125, no. 09, 2017, pp. 618–624., doi:10.1055/s-0043-101700.

Longo, Valter D., and Satchidananda Panda. "Fasting, Circadian Rhythms, and Time-Restricted Feeding in Healthy

Lifespan." *Cell Metabolism*, vol. 23, no. 6, 2016, pp. 1048–1059., doi:10.1016/j.cmet.2016.06.001.

Marinac, Catherine R., et al. "Prolonged Nightly Fasting and Breast Cancer Prognosis." *JAMA Oncology*, vol. 2, no. 8, 2016, p. 1049., doi:10.1001/jamaoncol.2016.0164

Michalsen A, Li C. 2013. *Fasting therapy for treating and preventing disease-current state of evidence.* Epub 2013 Dec 16.

Moro, Tatiana, et al. "Effects of Eight Weeks of Time-Restricted Feeding (16/8) on Basal Metabolism, Maximal Strength, Body Composition, Inflammation, and Cardiovascular Risk Factors in Resistance-Trained Males." *Journal of Translational Medicine*, vol. 14, no. 1, 2016, doi:10.1186/s12967-016-1044-0.

Patterson, Ruth E., and Dorothy D. Sears. "Metabolic Effects of Intermittent Fasting." *Annual Review of Nutrition*, vol. 37, no. 1, 2017, pp. 371–393., doi:10.1146/annurev-nutr-071816-064634.

Strong, James. *The Exhaustive Concordance of the Bible:* (electronic ed.) Woodside Bible Fellowship. Ontario 1996

Weil Andrew. 2012. *Intermittent Fasting: A Healthy Choice.* Huffington Post

Wilcoxson, Jannie. 2007. *The Word on Health and Nutrition*